Recipes for Elevation
By
Ra Sekhi Arts Temple

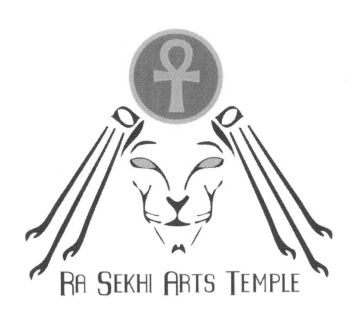

Table of Contents

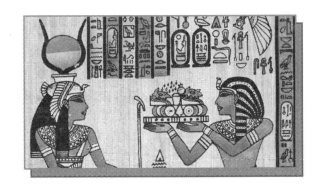

Preface

The recipes contained in this book are offered by healers: members of the Ra Sekhi Temple, founded by Queen Mother Rekhit Kajara Nia Yaa Nebthet. We are masters and practitioners of Ra Sekhi Kemetic Reiki. The purpose of this book is threefold. One purpose is to offer a range of vegetarian, vegan and raw food recipe ideas, as well as natural remedies for common ailments and information about nutritious foods. Another purpose is to assist those who wish to transition into vegetarianism, a vegan or a raw food diet. The most important purpose of this book, as the title implies, is to offer recipes for food that elevates. What does this mean?

Quantum physics tells us that everything in the omniverse vibrates and has its own frequency. Food has vibration levels. If you feel sleepy or lethargic (sluggish) after you have eaten, chances are you have consumed a food of low vibration. Conversely, if after eating a meal you feel full of sekhem (life force energy), you have probably eaten food of high vibration. Foods of the highest vibration are those that absorb maximum energy from the sun and the least from the earth. They are etheric foods—they elevate consciousness. Examples of these are tree fruits, nuts (cashews, walnuts and almonds grow high on trees) and coconuts, water that is clean and pure, clean air and sunlight. Yes, sunlight. Sunlight is a primary source of the very important vitamin

Next highest in energy are ground foods. They grow closest to the earth and get more energy from the earth than the sun. They are nutrient-rich and easily assimilated by the body. Leafy green vegetables, which contain sun-absorbing chlorophyll, and green beans, are examples that fall into this category, along with broccoli and zucchini. These foods also cleanse the body.   The least high in vibration are the foods that grow below ground, the earth foods. These foods get a huge amount of energy from the earth, and sun energy indirectly. Some examples of these are carrots, beets, parsnips, garlic, yams and onions. Though lower in vibration than ground and sun foods, these root vegetables can be very healing.

Eating high vibration food enables us to be more in tune with the Divine Source. You've probably heard "Your body is your temple" and "You are what you eat". As a light being having a human experience, your body is where the Divine Source dwells. The Divine Source is not outside of us but within us. When low vibration foods and processed foods are eaten and overeaten, it eventually leads to illnesses which distract us from connecting with the Most High within us. We ruin the temple that holds our divinity. In addition, low vibration foods result in an imbalance of our emotions and inhibit our ability to focus. This, in turn, may affect our behavior in ways that do not serve us. The Almighty One has created all naturally growing foods to serve us, sustain us and maintain us by infusing them with what we need for optimal health and vitality. Let us, in turn, endeavor to acknowledge the divine within us by ensuring that our body temples vibrate at the highest of frequencies.

--Mut Shat Shemsut--

Food Facts

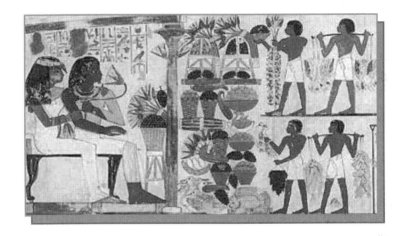

Balancing the Blood

The old saying "you are what you eat " applies even more when we overstand the importance of having alkaline blood. We should eat foods that will keep our alkaline/acid balanced in our blood. When the blood is more alkaline it is difficult for dis-ease to live in one's body. When the blood is more alkaline the body is in harmony and organs can function the way they are meant to. These lists are meant to assist you in learning the science of food. For best results eat a wide variety of fresh fruits and vegetables and grains everyday.

Very Alkaline Forming

Alfalfa grass (lucerne)
Barley grass
Beet greens
Bok choy
Chard
Collards
Dandelion greens
Figs
Green juices
Kale
Lemons
Limes
Leafy greens (most)
Spinach
Watercress
Miso
Olives
Oranges
Papaya
Parsley
Seaweed
Sea vegetables
Watermelon

Slightly Alkaline Forming

Almonds
Amaranth
Artichoke
Brussel sprouts
Buckwheat (sprouted)
Flaxseeds
Lentils (sprouted)
Millet
Mushrooms
Olive oil
Potato (with skins)
Pumpkin seeds
Quinoa
Sesame seeds
Sprouted grains (possibly neutral)
Sprouted seeds
Sunflower seeds
Wild rice

Alkaline forming Foods

Apples
Apricots
Avocado
Bananas
Beet root
Bell pepper
Berries (most)
Blackberries
Broccoli
Cabbage
Carob
Carrots
Cauliflower
Cayenne pepper
Chlorella (some)
Celery
Cherries
Chive
Cilantro
Corn (sweet)
Cucumber
Currants
Dates
Daikon
Eggplant
Endive
Garlic
Ginger root
Grapes
Grapefruit
Green beans
Green herbs
Guava
Kohlrabi

Kiwi fruit
Leeks
Lettuce
Mango
Mangosteen
Melons
Mustard greens
Nectarines
Okra
Onions
Parsnip
Passion fruit
Peaches
Pears
Peppers
Persimmons
Pineapple
Prickley pear
Pumpkin
Raisins
Raspberry
Rutabaga
Sapote
Spirulina (some)
Sprouts
Strawberries
Squash
Sweet potato
Tangerines
Taro root
Tomato
Turnip
Young coconut
Zucchini

Acid Forming Foods
Cranberries (slightly)
Blueberries (slightly)
Plums (slightly)
Prunes (slightly)
Unripe fruit
Most nuts and seeds
Fermented foods
Processed fruit juices (store bought)
Peanuts
Soft drinks
Alcoholic beverages
Dairy
Meat
Most grains
Most beans
Processed foods

Some acidic foods can be helpful, like lemons and other cit-rus fruit. Some acidic substances can be very harmful, like soda, which if consumed too much can lead to tooth decay, nervous issues, arthritis and many more physical ailments. It is said it will take 8 glasses of water to restore your blood level after drinking 1 (12 ounce) soft drink/soda. Imagine the effects of that acid in your body if you drink more soda than water. The preservatives To keep your energy and vi-tality high consume less acidic foods and more alkaline food. See yourself as a divine temple and make a commitment to give yourself and your family the best food possible.

Vitality Tips

Pineapple

Pineapples can add a nice tropical flair to any smoothie. However, there is more to this spiny looking fruit than meets the eye. Not only does it contain manganese, which aids in healthy bone development, but also has properties that act as an anti-inflammatory on painfully swollen joints. Needless to say, pineapples are great for arthritis. It can also be helpful in providing vitamin C and reducing mucus and sinus fluid during cold, flu, or sinusitis bouts.

Mango

This fruit tastes so good, give thanks that it is so good for you! The mango alkalizes the whole body! It's the tartaric, malic and citric acids that do this work. According to researchers, the antioxidants found in mangoes have been found to protect against leukemia, colon, prostate and breast cancers. The pectin, vitamin C and fiber content of the mango helps to lower bad cholesterol—Low Density Lipopro-tein). Mangoes clear the skin from within, and can also be used topically to clear pimples (which you won't get if you eliminate dairy, processed and fried foods!) and unclog pores. Mangoes also protect the eyes against night blindness and dry eyes via its Vitamin A content.

Coconut

The coconut is referred to as a "functional food" because it has so many health benefits. Another power food, you may consume it and use it on my hair and skin as well. Calcium, iron, copper, zinc and selenium are just a few of the minerals coconut contains. B-6, B-12, riboflavin, E and Retinol are just a few of the vitamins. It also contains a vitamin called pantothenic acid (B-5), which is found in every cell of the body and in all living things. Among other attributes, it helps heal wounds, balance cholesterol, and make-up for other vitamin deficiencies.

Strange Fruit?

Avocados can be used as a really great base for a smoothie, especially if dairy isn't your thing or you want to transition from vegetarianism to veganism. Ripe avocados add a smooth creamy texture to your favorite smoothie without sacrificing flavor. Not only are great for your heart & reproductive organs, but full of vitamins such as K & E.

Give Herbs a Chance

Cilantro is a powerful little herb with a citrus like flavor with a hint of pepper. It is jam packed with vitamins & minerals and helps to lower bad cholesterol and regulate heart rate and blood pressure. Throw a few leaves in your smoothie for a zesty flavorful surprise.

All Hail Kale!

Kale comes from the same family of vegetables as broccoli, cabbage, and cauliflower. It has nearly double the calcium of spinach and a remarkable amount of fiber for a leafy green vegetable. Like many other green vegetables, it contains many cancer-fighting phytonutrients along with vitamins and minerals great for the bones and eyes.

Coconut Oil

As you may already know, coconut oil is a wonderful source of natural energy. When choosing a coconut oil one may wonder what the difference is between unrefined and refined. Refined oils are more processed and have been bleached and deodorized. Refined oils are generally considered cleaner and safer for raw consumption. Unrefined coconut oil is considered crude because it contains more of the fruits natural essence and generally has not had heat applied throughout the production process. Not only is the flavor and aroma of coconut more evident it contains more nutrients than its refined counterpart.

Peachy Clean!

In some cultures, peaches are used to detoxify and cleanse unhealthy kidneys. In addition to aiding with kidney function peaches have been known to assist with healthy digestion. This juicy fruit is also antioxidant; full of vitamins and minerals like vitamin A, potassium, and calcium.

Want a thicker smoothie?

Try using frozen fruit instead of ice for a thicker, richer smoothie. You can always use any liquid of choice such as fruit juice, water, milk, etc. to tone it down if necessary while adding another dimension of flavor.

You are what you eat!

Did you know that celery consists of 23% of sodium just like your bones? Not only does celery resemble the bones it is also good for providing nutrients to them. Other bone-like vegetables such as rhubarb are also great as well.

Food that Protect the Eyes--Have it for the Eyes!

Below is a list of foods that protect the eyes, you will find recipes that use them in the book. With the absence of these foods in the diet and prolonged computer use, we compromise our vision. These foods work for us!

Apricots—good for night vision—contains beta carotene that the body converts to vitamin A—the eye vitamin.

Carrots, sweet potatoes, cantaloupe and winter squash also contain beta carotene

Coconut milk yogurt—rich and creamy, like dairy yogurt it usually contains an active bacterial culture (Good bacteria, of course!), but not always, so check the label.

Try these other fruits in muffins: Oranges, peaches, strawberries, tomatoes, and red bell peppers help support blood vessels in the eye and may reduce risk of cataracts.

Resources:nuts.com

Personal Products

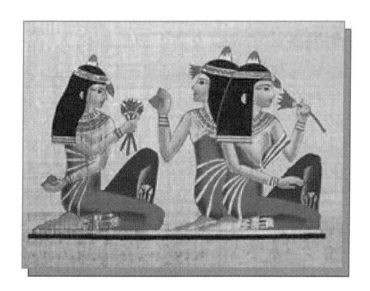

Body Butter

By Nia Yaa

1 lb shea butter

1 cup coconut oil

1/4 cup of beeswax

1/2 cup of almond oil

1/2 cup of lavender flowers

Directions

Add lavender to almond oil on very low heat. Simmer for 20 minutes then take the flowers out with a spoon. Add shea butter and coconut oil. Let simmer and mix well. Let the mix cool and pour into glass jars to store. Add lavender oil when the blend begins to solidify. Add more beeswax if you want butter to be thicker

I have made this for my family for over twenty years, it is good to protect, nourish, moisturize and heal skin and hair.

Herbal Massage Oil

By Nia Yaa

3/4 cup of jojoba or almond oil

1/2 tsp of essential rose oil

1/2 tsp of essential lavender oil

1/2 tsp of essential geranium oil

1/2 tsp of essential ylang-ylang oil

Directions

Mix together, shake well and store in a tightly sealed dark glass container. Use for massage, add 2 teaspoons to your bath or apply to your pulse points.

Tooth powder

By Nia Yaa

1/4 cup baking soda

1/3 cup of bentonite clay

1 tsp myrrh powder

3 –7 drops essential peppermint oil

3-7 drops of anise oil (optional)

Directions

Mix well and store in a glass jar. Use in the morning and evening for best results.

Glycerin soap

By Nia Yaa

1 lb of glycerin melt and pour soap

1/2 cup of clay

Essential oil

Directions

Melt glycerin on low heat. When melted mix in clay and stir well. Pour into mold and let cool. Add drops of oil to molds before it cools. Lavender, frankincense, sage, peppermint , etc.

When you make your own products you control what you put on and in your body.

Aloe face scrub

By Nia Yaa

2 tbsp. of aloe gel

2 tsp of oatmeal

1 tsp of sea salt

Distilled or filtered water

Directions

Mix ingredients. Add enough water to make a paste. Massage onto face and throat. Leave on for five to ten minutes. Rinse with cool water. Repeat once a week to heal blemishes.

Salt Body Scrub

By Nia Yaa

1/4 cup of sea salt

1/4 cup of coconut or cold pressed olive oil

1 tbsp lavender flowers

1 tbsp. rose flowers

Directions

Mix ingredients.

Massage onto body with hands or mitt.

Affirmation : My skin is healthy and glowing.

Seed Scrub

By Nia Yaa

1/2 cup ground oatmeal

1/3 cup ground sunflower seeds

4 tbsp. almond meal

1 tsp ground rosemary

Distilled or filtered water*

Directions

Mix dry ingredients well and store in a jar. When ready to use add about 2 tsps. Of dry mix to enough water to make a smooth paste. Allow to thicken then spread on face or body. Leave on for ten minutes then rinse with warm water.

*Coconut milk may be substituted for water for dry skin.

Herbal Body Wash

By Nia Yaa

1/2 cup of black soap

1 tsp of almond or grapeseed oil

5 drops each of tea tree, peppermint, lemon

water

Directions

Add ingredients to a jar and fill with water. Shake well and let sit until soap melts. Pour into plastic soap bottle when ready to use.

Affirmation: Lovingly prepared...lovingly received

Herbal eye rinse

By Nia Yaa

2 tbsp. eyebright

2 tbsp. of chamomile

2 cups distilled water

Directions

Bring water to a boil and remove from heat. Add herbs, cover and steep for about 1 hour. Strain and store in glass bottle. Splash or mist eyes to refresh tired eyes. Refrigerate and discard after 7 days.

Herbal insect repellent

By Nia Yaa

2 cups witch hazel

1 tsp of citronella essential oil

1 tsp of lemon essential oil

1 tsp of red vinegar

Directions

Combine ingredients in a bowl or jar.

Add to a spray bottle, apply as needed.

Baby's Soothing Teething Gum Relief

By Aura Agape

In a small clean container with lid, add the following ingredients:

1 tbs Organic Cold-Pressed Extra Virgin Olive Oil

1 drop Clove Essential Oil

Directions

Mix ingredients together to dilute and add to cotton swab or directly to fingers and apply to effected area on the gums for relief. Many cranky babies return to happy ones after using this remedy.

Herbs'N Natural Gargle and Mouthwash

By Aura Agape

For relieving sore & scratchy throats, mouth sores, removing mucus, plaque and other debris from the mouth:

gargle with salt water. 1 tsp salt with 1 cup of warm water.

Another recipe calls for ¼ tsp Myrrh Gum resin to be steeped in 1 cup of hot water for 10 minutes and allowed to cool for another 5-10 minutes. Strain the tea and swish and gargle to relieve mouth sores and even sore throat caused by infection such as strep throat.

Myrrh is useful for bleeding gums, gingivitis, tonsillitis, sore throat (including strep throat), and bronchitis. Note: This is a bitter herb but, it works so well, you will appreciate it.

Affirmation: I speak with love, joy and kindness.

Garlic Oil for Earache Relief

By Aura Agape

When the little one is fussy and pulling at the ear, it may be possible that there is an ear infection. I have heard some mothers say that they can smell the ear infection others just know the signs such as pain, earache, headache, sore throat, fever, congestion, irritability, runny nose, tinnitus and vertigo. It is wise to have a qualified practitioner to see if it is indeed an ear infection and rule out anything more serious or if a more aggressive or alternate treatment is necessary. In general, this remedy works well on children and adults alike.

Heat a small pan on mid-low setting and add the following ingredients:

6 tbs Organic Cold-Pressed Extra Virgin Olive Oil

1 large crushed garlic clove

Allow oil to heat slowly until the fragrance of the garlic is noticeable. Garlic should gently simmer in oil for 10-15 minutes.

Allow to cool to a safe temperature for delicate skin. Strain using a cheese cloth or simply remove the garlic clove from the oil and pour into 2oz dropper bottle or any small clean jar with lid.

Optional Ingredients: Add 2 drops of Lavender Essential oil and 1 drop of Thyme essential oil to handle chronic ear infections. Use a clean cotton ball, tear a piece that is small enough to fit into the outer portion of the ear canal and saturate with the oil and apply. Alternatively I add a few drops

into the ear and gently insert a small piece of cotton into the entrance of the ear canal to make sure that the oil gets to the middle ear to offer relief.

Abscess Control

(Anti-Microbial Powder for Tooth, Gums and Mouth)

By Aura Agape

When a tooth/teeth get one or multiple cavities, or a condition forms where dental work is needed and long overdue, it is common that at some point, and infection may occur. If infection gets to be out of control, an abscess may form, it can be very painful while causing swelling due to inflammation, pus and fluid build-up.

1/8 tsp Myrrh Gum Powder

1/8 tsp Golden Seal Root Powder

1/8 tsp Turmeric Root Powder

1 drop clove oil

1 tsp Organic Cold-Pressed Extra Virgin Olive Oil

Directions

Mix the dry ingredients together and dip a clean cotton ball or gauze in the oil. Follow up by dusting the cotton ball or gauze with the herbal powder mix. Make sure to get good coverage as the herbs should lay against the sore and infected area(s) in the mouth along the gum line. Change throughout the day as necessary.

This offers pain relief, reduces swelling and speeds the recovery process. Positive results can range from a few hours to a few days in more serious cases and in the elderly. In all cases, an abscess is an indication that there is a serious underlying problem. Proper, consistent oral care is a must! Due to the sensitivity of the mouth, it is wise to be gentle while cleaning. Food and drink should be taken in on the opposite side of the mouth. Swishing with Salt-Water gargle should clear the mouth of food and beverage particles and help to kill the germs in the mouth in before application. This remedy only offers temporary relief until you can reach your dentist.

Spiritual Baths

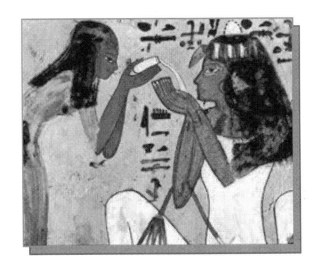

Gemstones and the Spiritual Bath
By Mut Shat Shemsut

For years I was a shower girl. Always in a hurry, baths just seemed too time-consuming. Even when I had time to take one, the shower seemed more hygienic. I have since trans- formed myself into a woman who appreciates the power of the bath. As I went through the gateways with Queen Afua, and using her book, *Sacred Woman* as a guide, I rediscov- ered the pleasure of immersion in water, which I had actually loved and appreciated as a child. Now, though, instead of bubble bath, it's herbs, aromas, ambiance—and gemstones. Below is one of my favorite recipes for a spiritual, healing bath.

2 teabags of hyssop or 2 tbs. of the loose herbs
2 teabags of milk thistle or 2 tbs. of the loose herbs
Florida water
Hyssop oil
½ cup of sea salt
Sage for burning
One 8 lb clear quartz crystal
Rose quartz
Clear quartz crystal clusters
Your favorite incense
three white candles
uplifting music

Have your favorite incense burning in the bathroom, close the door.
Have uplifting music playing.
Put over a quart of water to boil
Run your bath water.
Place the tea bags in the jar; pour the boiling water over them; leave some room at the top
(I usually let the teas sit overnight)
Add three or four drops of Florida water
Add ½ cup of sea salt
Smudge your bathroom with the sage
Place three lit candles (white) in a triangle formation around the tub, so that you would sit at its base
Place the 8 lb crystal quartz in the tub
Place the rose quartz and crystal quartz clusters around your tub

Shake your tea mixture; pour a quarter of it in the bath; as you pour, give thanks to The Source, our Creator. Ask that the bath you are about to take be a healing bath, healing your mind, your body, and your spirit. Ask that any negativity within your body temple or your space be removed.
Add three or four drops of the hyssop oil
Luxuriate
You may want to pray for healing during your bath.

Note: Rose quartz is a wonderful, powerful stone that has heart-healing properties that bathe the body, mind and spirit in its healing and enlightening love frequency. Clear quartz crystal resonates with all the chakras. It also amplifies the energies of other stones. It can be programmed with positive thoughts and feelings. Both stones have other attributes as well.

You can place other stones in your bath that address just about any concern. For example, amethyst dissolves anger, lepidolite helps to remove doubt, lepidolite and moonstone encourage feelings of balance.   Two of many excellent books for understanding more about gem stones are Rocks of Ages: Anu Edition by Ras Ben and The Book of Stones by Robert Simmons and Naisha Ahsian.

Two of my favorite CDs for some serious healing are *Himalayan Chakra Healing* by Paradiso & Suren Shrestha and *The Heart of Healing* by Mirabai Ceiba. Other CDs that keep me feeling light are by Earth, Wind and Fire and Al Jarreau.

Spiritual Bath- Khepera Enhancer

By Aqseshsha Asu-At

Materials:

Big Glass or Metal bowl/container

Water (Spring, river, ocean water is good but optional)

7 drops Lavender oil

3 drops Sweet Orange oil

Dried or fresh roses or assorted flowers including roses

Rose Quartz Crystal

Amethyst Crystal

Sea Salt

1/2 tsp Florida water

Let your spirit guide!

Directions

Fill bowl with water and add the ingredients one by one making sure to mix the ingredients well with your hands and stating your positive intentions. This spiritual bath is great for repelling negative energy in the form of depression, sadness, and feelings of hopelessness. It helps to draw in the energy of universal love filling your heart and mind with peace, love, and ecstatic joy. This is also a great mix to add to a relaxing candlelit bath. Go ahead and do something kind for yourself!

Affirmation: I am happy, healthy and whole.

Uplifting Spiritual Bath

By Nia Yaa

This bath is perfect for those dealing with depression or stress. It will lighten your spirit and refresh your aura.

3 red roses or dried rose petals

3 carnations (yellow or white)

2 tblsp of lavender flowers

4 tblsp of sea salt

2 tblsp of baking soda

7 drops of jasmine oil

7 drops of frankincense oil

1 blue candle

Jasmine or lavender incense

1 amethyst crystal

Directions

Take petals off of the flowers. Add ingredients to a natural container with enough water to cover mixture. Crush flower petals with your hands while saying your prayers. Pour mixture directly into tub of lukewarm water. Light candle and incense. Soak and sing for 20—30 minutes. Make sure to submerge yourself three times to clear your entire aura. Think about the things that make you happy while in the tub. Cover yourself in white and sit quietly after the bath. This bath can be repeated once a week or until you feel lighter.

Qamarah's Free Flow Spiritual Bath
By Qamarah Muhammah El Shamesh

Spring water
Fresh flowers (let spirit guide)
Crystals (your choice)
Your choice of herbs ie. lavender
Clear Vodka or Florida water
bergamot essential oil
Lavender essential oil
Prayers
Tibetan singing bowl tunes
Love

Pour mixed ingredients in bottles or a gallon jug

Use during your shower time

Feel your aura strength

Be light & Free!

Spiritual Wash for the Home
By Nia Yaa

1/3 cup of baking soda
1/3 cup of sea salt
1 tsp cinnamon
7 drops frankincense oil
7 drops lavender oil
3 dashes of florida water
Directions

Add ingredients to a large bucket. Mix well and add your words of power to the bath. Use to wash your floors, walls and baseboards. Keep your thoughts and intentions clear as your clean your house. Make sure to wash the physical dirt before doing this cleanse. It will help raise the energy in your home. Use as often as you like.

Peaceful Blessings

Smoothies, Teas & Tonics

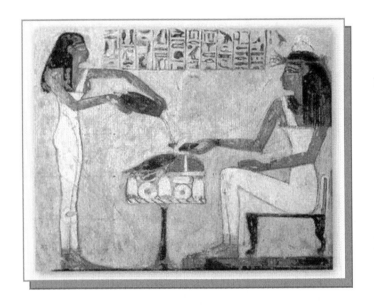

Herb'N Spice Tea

By Aura Agape

Whenever a loved one or myself is not feeling well, I am usually able to find helpful herbs in the kitchen that help to make it all better. Usually the change of seasons such as winter to spring and summer to fall bring about a change that trigger allergies, asthma, other respiratory and skin reactions.

When I am dealing with sinus congestion, I reach for a handful/4tbs of dried Rosemary to steep in approx. 2qts of near-boiling water for approx. 15 minutes. This recipe can be modified to suit the needs of the recipient.

Many times sinus infections can cause post-nasal drip and move to the lungs. To remedy this, I like to reach for a small handful of sprigs or 2tbs of dried Thyme and add to the above mixture. Basil can be added in the same fashion for relaxing bronchioles and expelling mucus. Strain leaves and add to lemonade or the juice of about 4-5 lemons and top off with enough water to fill 2 qt container. Optional: Add your choice of raw sugar, honey, agave, maple syrup or stevia to taste. Serve warm or chilled. Drink 3 cups a day.

1 handful each of Rosemary leaves and Nettles.

2 tbs each Thyme, and Basil

2 quart water for steeping & add more to top off the evaporated water during the boiling and steeping process.

Natural sweetener of choice such as: raw agave, raw honey*, raw sugar, maple syrup, or Stevia (Optional).

Note: Ratios for measuring Raw & Dried herbs are 3:1. Dried herbs are considered more potent due to the higher concentrations of essential oils.

Blood Tonic

By Nia Yaa

2 tbsp. hibiscus

2 tbsp. red clover

2 tbsp. raw ginger grated

1 tsp cinnamon

1 tsp cloves

1 dash of cayenne pepper

Directions

Add ingredients to large pot of water. Bring water to boil then simmer for 10 minutes. Let sit for 1 hour or more before drinking. This tea can be served warm or cold. Drink 3 times a day for best results.

Add 2 tbsp. blackstrap molasses for iron boost. Add honey or agave to sweeten if you like.

Cold Remedy

By Nia Yaa

1/2 onion

3 cloves garlic

1 med piece ginger

2 tblsp burdock

2 tblsp hibiscus

2 tblsp elderberries

1 tsp goldenseal

Directions

Add ingredients to large pot of water. Bring to a boil for 5 minutes. Then turn down fire and simmer for 20 minutes. Let sit for at least 1 hour before drinking. Add 1 tsp cayenne, 1 lemon and 2 tbsp. blackstrap molasses. Stir well then drink 3 times a day. Refrigerate after 24 hours.

Healers Cranberry Cleanse

By Qamarah Muhammad EL-Shamesh

Cranberries are an antioxidant powerhouse, so get them fresh during the fall and winter. By drinking this Healing Cranberry Cleanser green smoothie your body will experience the immediate effects of natural energy. Get your healthy dose of vitamin C and fiber in this healing green smoothie!

2 cups spinach, fresh

1 cup water

1 cup cranberries

2 oranges, peeled

2 bananas

. Serves 2 .

Directions

Blend spinach and water until smooth. Next add the remaining fruits and blend again.

* Use at least one frozen fruit to make the green smoothie cold.

TIP: Keep as much of the orange pith (the white part) on to add nutritional benefits.

Affirmation: I am free from all toxins and dis-ease.

Strawberry Passion

By Aqseshsha Asu-At

1 Frozen Banana

1c Frozen strawberries

1c Raw Spinach

2 TBS of Peanut Butter

1/4c uncooked steel cut oatmeal

1/2c Almond Milk

1/4c of Water

1Tbs of Agave Nectar or Grade B Maple syrup optional

Blend and enjoy

Strawberry Lemonade Bliss

By Qamarah Muhammad EL-Shamesh

10 strawberries

1 lemon, juiced

4 dates (or 2 tbs raw honey)

1tablespoon Chia seed (if desired)

1tablespoon Organic Maca

I quart pure water

Blend well.

Serves 3

Berry Kiwi Blast

By Qamarah Muhammad EL-Shamesh

Berries are naturally sweet immunity boosters, low-calorie, and full of antioxidants.

Kiwi is packed with vitamin C and an amazing fat-burning citrus fruit. I always keep several bags of frozen berries in the freezer.

2 cups spinach, fresh

2 cups water

1 cup blueberries*

1 cup mixed berries*

1 banana*

1 kiwi

1/2 avocado

– Serves 2 –

Directions

Blend spinach and water until smooth. Next add the remaining fruits and blend again.

Tip: Blend in 2 tablespoons of chia seeds or sprinkle on top.

Affirmation: Life-giving foods supply my body with all that it needs

Great Awakenings

By Aqseshsha Asu-At

1 c frozen fruit (strawberries, peaches, grapes, & melons)

½ c of spinach

1/4c Arugula

1/2c Almond Milk

1/2c Water

1TB raw coco powder

1tsp lemon juice

1Tbsp Agave nectar or grade B Maple Syrup

¼ c uncooked steel cut oats

1 Tbsp coconut oil

Directions

Blend and enjoy!

Queen's Nectar

by BarbaRa Sashemnu

One cup of almond milk or coconut milk

1/2 banana

1-2 scoops of whey protein

1/2 cup of berries (your choice)

One tbsp of Flax meal

Directions

Blend and enjoy

Sweeten to taste

Be the change you want to see

Htp

Strawberry Banana Smoothie with a Twist!

By Aqseshsha Asu-At

1 Frozen Chopped Banana

½ c Frozen Strawberries

1 c Kale

1Tbsp Raw Peanut Butter

1/2 c Coconut Milk

1 Tbsp Agave Nectar or Grade B Maple Syrup

1/4 c Water

Directions

Blend and enjoy!

Weed Seed Smoothie

By BarbaRa Sashemnu

Kale

One cup of blueberries

One ripe avocado

1/4 cup of Hemp seeds

2 tablespoon of Acai powder

One cup of pomegranate juice

2 tbsp Isofem whey protein

Directions

Blend and Enjoy

Affirmation: This drink is restoring my body, mind & soul.

Put the Lime in the Coconut

By Aqseshsha Asu-At

½ c Frozen Strawberries

½ c Frozen Melon

1 Avocado

1/2 c Coconut Milk

1 tsp Lime Juice

1 Tbsp of Agave Nectar or Grade B Maple syrup

Directions

Blend and enjoy

My favorite smoothie

By Nia Yaa

1 banana

1 cup fresh or frozen strawberries

1/2 cup blueberries

1 cup pineapple

1/4 cup coconut

1/4 cup goji berries

1 tbsp. chia seeds

1 tbsp. flax seeds

Add 4-6 cups of filtered water

Directions

Blend and enjoy

KISS (Keep it Simple Smoothie)

By Aqseshsha Asu-At

1 Frozen medium chopped banana

1/4 c Frozen Mango

1/4 c Frozen Pineapple

1/2 c Spinach

1/4 c Celery

1/2 Avocado

3/4 cup Apple Juice

1/4 c Water

Directions

Blend and enjoy

Power smoothie

By Nia Yaa

1 banana

1 cup fresh berries

1 mango

1/2 cup coconut

2 tbsp. blackstrap molasses

1/4 cup chia seeds

2 tbsp moringa

2 tbsp. spirulina

Add 4 cups of filtered water

Directions

Blend and enjoy

Mango Plantain Smoothie

By Mut Shat Shemsut

1 very ripe plantain (It should be black but not rotting!)

1 large mango

1 green organic apple

2 cups coconut water (or liquid of your choice)

1 tsp Queen Afua's Formula I Green Life*

1 tsp chia seeds

1 tsp spirulina

1 tsp chlorella

Directions

Peel and cut the mango fruit from the seed

Peel and cut up the apple

Pour in the coconut water

Drop all ingredients into a blender

Blend until smooth

- Queen Afua's Formula I Green Life contains wheatgrass, lecithin, psyllium husk and spirulina to enhance memory, the immune system and brain function.

Watermelon Ginger Snap

By Mut Shat Shemsut

This is a cool recipe for a warm day.

Ingredients

Chunks of black-seeded watermelon to fill a blender (remove seeds)

Mango or other fruit of your choice

2 heaping tbs of fresh shredded ginger

Directions

Blend the watermelon. Add more until the blender is ¾ filled

with watermelon juice. Cut mango away from the seed. Shred ginger. Add the mango and ginger to the watermelon juice. Blend.

Drink. Enjoy!

Affirmation: Good food is the key to my good health

Salads, Snacks & Sides

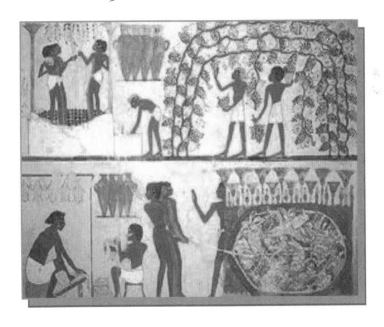

Summer Fruit Salad

By Nia Yaa

1/2 pineapple

1 apple

2 banana

1 mango

3 kiwi

1 cup of blueberries

10 strawberries

1 orange

Dash of cinnamon

Dash of honey or agave

Directions

Cut fruit. Mix well and serve

Winter Fruit Salad

By Nia Yaa

2 apples

2 pears

2 oranges

1/2 cup of coconut

1/2 cup of walnuts

1/2 cup of raisins or dried cranberries

Directions

Chop fruit, add a dash of honey or agave. Mix well and serve.

Sweet carrot salad

By Nia Yaa

2 cups of carrot pulp
1/2 chopped apple
1/2 cup of dried cranberries
1/2 cup of crushed walnuts
1/4 cup of chopped red onion
1/4 cup of chopped bell pepper
1/4 cup of olive oil
1/4 cup of balsamic vinegar
1/4 cup of honey or agave
1 dash of cinnamon and cumin
Directions

Mix well and chill before serving.

Watermelon Wave Salad

By Mut Shat Shemsut

1 medium-sized black seeded watermelon
2 mangoes
2 peaches
1 cup of shredded coconut
Directions

Cut watermelon up into small squares. Cut mangoes up into small pieces. Cut peaches up into small pieces.

Spoon all ingredients into a large bowl. Mix gently, you don't want to mash.

Sprinkle in shredded coconut.

Gently mix some more.

Serve

Chia Seed Banana Pudding Mix it Up

By Mut Shat Shemsut

Chia seeds are good for you. They are a superfood. They contain healthy omega-3 fatty acids, protein, fiber, carbohydrates, antioxidants and calcium. Unlike flaxseeds, chia seeds are an unprocessed, wholegrain food that can be absorbed by the body. These are the same seeds you saw in the Chia Pet/Obama bust commercials. Sprinkle in smoothies, on cereal, over vegetables, in sauces just about everything. If you are a vegan who misses yogurt and puddings and especially your mother's southern banana pudding with the vanilla wafers—this recipe is for you.

Ingredients

2 very ripe organic yellow bananas

6 tbs chia seeds

1 ½ cups of coconut, hemp or almond milk

¼ tsp organic vanilla

Directions

Mash up the bananas in a cereal size bowl. Add the coconut, hemp or almond milk. Mix it up. Spoon the chia seeds into the bowl. Mix it up. Add the vanilla. Mix it up.

Let it sit overnight.

The chia seed pudding will have a nice, thick consistency in the morning.

With Mama Nature's gift of fruit of every variety, the kinds of puddings you can make with chia seeds is almost limitless.

Tomato and Onion Goddess Dressing

By The Honey Diva

1 roasted tomato

1 small onion

1 garlic clove

1 1/2 Tbsp tahini

2 Tbsp of Nayonaise

1 Tbsp water

1/2 Tbsp lemon juice

1 1/2 tsp. Braggs liquid aminos

1 tsp olive oil

1 Tbsp of Honey

Bake the tomato, garlic and the onion for 20 minutes on 275 f. Peel the skin of tomato, add with onion and garlic to blender. Blend until you get a thin consistency. Add to a bowl and whisk all the ingredients in a small bowl. This will provide enough dressing for two very large salads.

Zesty Sandwich Spread

By Herb 'N Spice

1 tsp horseradish

1 tsp mustard

1 tsp barbeque sauce

1 tsp vegannaise

Directions

Mix together and use as a sandwich spread or dipping sauce.

Mama Dorothy's Salad Drizzle / Marinade
By Nova Kafele

2 1/2 cups Mothers Apple Cider Vinegar or Red Wine Vinegar
3 cloves garlic
1 sprig rosemary finely minced
1 sprig oregano finely minced
1 sprig thyme finely minced
1 tsp paprika
1/2 tsp cayenne (preferably AfRAkan Bird)
1/2 tsp Spike
2 Tbsp extra virgin olive oil
1 Tbsp agave nectar or your preferred sweetener
Directions

Add all ingredients together in a glass measuring cup so the contents are easy to pour into salad dressing bottle. Cover with plastic wrap or lid and let ingredients marinate for a few hours before serving. Pour into salad dressing container and refrigerate. Enjoy Mama Dorothy's Drizzle on your salads, fresh veggies or as marinade for your veggies before grilling.

This blend has proven to increase a person's appetite and also activate sluggish bowels. Can double the recipe and play with measurements of ingredients to fit your palate.

Enjoy!

Affirmation: My cells are elevated to a higher vibration

Inhale the Kale Salad

By Empress Tabia "Khet Ra Maat"

Salad

A bunch of Kale (Curly or Purple)

1 Cucumber (diced)

Plum Tomatoes (sliced)

Walnuts

Cranberries (handful)

Juicy Dressing

¼ cup vinegar

¼ cup of olive oil

3 tbsp Veganaise of your choice

1 Lime

1 Lemon

3 tbsp of honey or Agave

Spike Seasoning (to taste)

Sea Salt (to taste)

Preparation:

Connect to the Kale as you rip the leaves from their stalks and hand-shred them.

Once you've made a nice 'bed' top with all remaining salad ingredients get your hands in there and undo the bed! Toss and turn until all ingredients are distributed evenly while drizzling and coating with combined juicy dressing.

Tell it you love it and ask it to love you and fill you with joy.

Yum!

Jerk Plantain Salad

By Empress Tabia "Khet Ra Maat"

Ingredients:

2 Fully Ripe Plantains (the blacka the betta)

1 medium-sized Red Pepper (diced)

1 medium-sized Green Pepper (diced)

1 Red onion (chopped)

2 Limes

2 Tsp Agave

½ Tsp Jerk Seasoning (Walkerswood or Grace's)

Pinch of Sea Salt

Preparation:

Chop all the plantains and veggies singing a sweet tune

Squeeze the juice of 1 fresh lime over your ingredients so far

Combine the juice of the remaining lime, agave, jerk seasoning and pinch of salt and then coat the veggies.

Serve chilled or at room temperature.

(Tip: Becomes perfectly marinated after a day or two)

Affirmation: Sweet foods give me sweet thoughts.

Plantain Salad I by Mut Shat Shemsut/Giamprem

2 ripe, sweet (yellow) plantains

½ red pepper

1 red onion

6 sprigs of parsley

4 or 5 light sprinkles of dulse

Directions

Slice plantains into medallions. Finely chop red onions. Finely chop or cut parsley. Toss everything around in a bowl. Sprinkle in the dulse. Toss again. Serves four.

Plantain Salad II

2 ripe, sweet plantains

2 cups couscous

3 cloves garlic

6 sprigs of parsley

1 Tbs coconut oil

Directions

Pour cous cous in a bowl, rinse it and "just" cover it with distilled water. Set aside.

Slice plantain into diagonals. Finely chop the garlic. Finely cut or chop the parsley. Toss everything around in a bowl. Add the couscous and olive oil.

Toss some more. Serves Four.

Why they're good for you...

Plantains—promote digestion, help body to retain more calcium, phosphorous, and nitrogen, which helps to rejuvenate healthy tissue; plantain sugar is easily metabolized; high levels of vitamin A, potassium, calcium, iron and finer; help to relieve constipation; low in sodium, no cholesterol.

Collard Green Salad

By Herb 'N Spice

½ bunch organic collard greens

1 cup shredded organic carrots, beets, turnips and, herbs like parsley, watercress,

or a few sprigs of cilantro

2-3 cloves garlic (minced) equivalent of 1 tbsp

1/3 organic apple cider vinegar

¼ organic extra virgin olive oil

3 tbsp raw agave nectar

1 tsp nutritional yeast

Pink Himalayan Sea Salt

Green Life Seasoning Spice Blend

Directions

½ bunch of collard greens (washed well & sliced thinly or torn into small bite-sized pieces). It is optional to add

shredded carrots, beets, turnips, or herbs like parsley, watercress, a few sprigs of cilantro...to the mix. Be creative and go for color! Colorful peppers will do just the trick. Add about a tbs of minced garlic (2-3 cloves) if you choose.

Mix well & sprinkle a tsp each of chia, flax or even sunflower or pumpkin seeds. I did an omega-3 rich combo of chia and flax seeds as an option. Serve, eat up and enjoy. It is even better if you let it sit overnight chilled to marinate.

Growing God/Goddess Salad with Mojito Dressing"

By Empress Tabia 'Khetera Ma'at'

1 bunch of Swiss Chard (or any leafy green of your choosing)

3 radishes (cleaned and sliced)

1/4 green bell pepper (diced or cubed)

1/4 red bell pepper (diced or cubed)

1 cucumber (diced or cubed)

Fistful of bean sprouts (mung bean or any sprouts of your choosing)

Fistful of cranberries

Dressing (Make in a glass jar to store, and add as you consume Goddess salad to preserve freshness*)

Palm-full of mint leaves (quickly shredded: use your hands)

1/4 green bell pepper (diced or cubed)

1/4 red bell pepper (diced or cubed)

1/4 c extra virgin olive oil

1/4 c distilled white vinegar

Juice of 1/2 lime or juice of 1 key lime

1-1 1/2 tbsp of agave nectar

1-1 1/2 tbsp of Chipotle Mayo Veganaise (Grapeseed could work)

Sea Salt and Spike Seasoning to taste

Directions

Shake up the dressing ingredients (Put your hips in it :-) For brothers, just shake with your biceps ;-))

Pour over Growing God/Goddess Salad *top with chopped nuts if you have any or aren't allergic.

Full Joy. Peace & Light

Tun-No Salad

By Herbs'N Spice

5-7 carrots

Small onion

Small firm and sweet apple

1 celery stick

1 tsp of minced garlic (2-3 cloves)

1 tbsp apple cider vinegar

Herb'N Spice Green Seasoning Blend *

Vegannaise (3-5 tbsp to desired consistency)

Directions

Juice 5-7 carrots depending on size (get enough pulp to equate a couple of cans of albacore tuna). Drink the juice but save the pulp and put in a bowl.

Dice a small onion. Cut a small apple in cubes. Dice 1 celery stick and add a tsp of garlic (optional). Add 1 tbs apple cider vinegar. Season with Herb'N Spice Green Seasoning

Blend or use your favorite seasoning and add extra seaweed (optional) for seafood flavor such as Kelp, Spirulina, Chlorella. Add about 3-5 heaping tbsp. of vegannaise and mix all together. You may use regular mayo but less will be required as regular mayo is more oily. I hope that you enjoy it. I add it to salads, wraps, on sprouted whole grain bread, or a whole grain cracker.

*Alternative to Herb'N Spice Green Life Spice Blend:

 Use your favorite all-purpose seasoning such as Herb'N Spice Original Blend and add 1/2tsp kelp/spirulina/chlorella (add more if you desire more of a fish flavor. 1 tbs nutritional yeast (optional).

Affirmation: I am so thankful for this divine meal.

Forbidden Rice Salad

By Herb 'N Spice

2 cups Black Rice

4 cups water

Sea Salt

1 med carrot

1 broccoli crown or bunch of fresh herbs

1 lemon

2 tbsp vegannaise

Directions

Cook 2 Cups Black Rice in 4 Cups Water. Add Sea Salt to taste (optional). Bring to boil and reduce to simmer 45 minutes or until tender. Add 1 med carrot diced or shredded. Chop broccoli crown or fresh herbs (i.e. parsley, mint leaves, etc...) add to rice. Squeeze fresh lemon juice over the mixture and add 2 tbsp Vegannaise. Mix ingredients & chill 30 minutes or more.

Spicy Guacamole

By Nia Yaa

2 avocado

1 jalapeno pepper

1 roma tomato

2 cloves of garlic

Lemon juice

Cayenne pepper

Directions

Mash avocado and add chopped tomato,pepper and garlic. Mix well , add lemon juice and cayenne to taste.

Not so Nutty Nut Sauce

By Mut Shat Shemsut

1tbsp of the sweetener of your choice (Suggestions: palm sugar, coconut sweetener)

¾ cups of almonds, sunflower seeds and hazelnuts (you don't have to use all three)

1 tsp of fresh cilantro, chopped

2 tsp of sundried tomato

4 tbsp of juice of 1 lime

¼ cup of room temperature purified water

Directions

Always soak your nuts and seeds overnight. Combine all solid ingredients in a food processor. Add lime juice. Drizzle in water if needed to thin almonds, sunflower seeds and hazelnuts all contain vitamin E and may hinder age-related macular degeneration.

Sprouting Quinoa

By Mut Shat Shemsut

To prepare raw quinoa sprouts, first rinse the seeds and soak them for at least eight hours. Each seed is coated with saponin, a natural insect repellent that can give quinoa a bitter taste if not removed by soaking. Next, drain the seeds, rinse three times and place in a jar that is kept in a warm location away from direct sunlight.

You will need to drain and re-rinse the quinoa three times daily for three days before the first edible shoots emerge. Use the raw quinoa sprouts on sandwiches or in stir fries and salads. Keep the sprouts in the refrigerator. Warning: Dispose of them promptly if you notice mold.

Quinoa lowers the glycemic-index which reduces the risk of age-related macular degeneration.

Note: Quinoa may be eaten raw as sprouts. However, if you're not going to follow the steps above, COOK IT!

For the Main Course

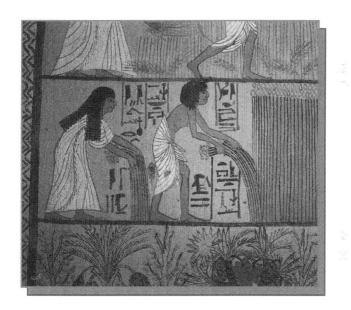

Brussel Sprouts, The Cabbage Mini-Me

By Mut Shat Shemsut

Brussels sprouts, with their tight green leaves, look like tiny cabbages. They should, they're related! Though tiny, they pack a lot of benefits. Brussels sprouts contain sulforaphane, which is believed to be a cancer fighter. They are best eaten raw in order to maintain the potency of that chemical. The vegetable also contains immune system boosting vitamin C, which is good for fighting colds and healing cuts.

Brussels Sprouts as a Main Dish

Ingredients

5 cups of sliced Brussels sprouts

1 cup of sun-dried tomatoes

2 tablespoons of fresh lemon juice

1 tsp of garlic

1 tablespoon of coconut or olive oil

½ cup of red onions

½ cup of red bell pepper

Pink Himalayan Sea Salt

Directions

Remove any yellowing or limp leaves, or leaves with holes.

Slice the Brussels sprouts. Place all ingredients in a food processor except the salt . Once ground, remove to bowl

Salt to taste

Serves 8

Goes well with a romaine lettuce and cucumber salad.

Raw Avocado Kale Pesto with Zucchini Noodles

(serves 4)

by Mama Annette Hurt

4 medium zucchini

1 cup cherry tomatoes, sliced in half

3-4 cloves garlic

2 avocados

1/4 cup cold pressed olive oil

1/4 cup nutritional yeast (optional)

1/2 cup pine nuts plus some for garnish

1 small bunch kale, de- stemmed and torn into small pieces

2 bunches basil

1 TB lemon juice

Directions

Pinch Himalayan salt and fresh cracked pepper

1.Shred zucchini in mandolin. Set aside in colander to drain excess liquid. (You may need to squeeze to remove excess water)

2.Start food processor running. Drop cloves of garlic in one at a time.

3.Add avocado, olive oil, nutritional yeast, pine nuts, and lemon juice. Pulse till blended.

4. Add kale and basil until well chopped and incorporated.

5. Season to taste with salt and pepper, then toss with zucchini noodles and tomatoes.

Affirmation: **I am cleansed, restored and strengthened with every bite/sip.**

Raw Spaghetti Squash

Both by Aqseshsha Asu-At

1 Spaghetti squash

1 medium tomato

3 cloves garlic

2 tbsp Nutritional Yeast

1/4 tsp Sea Salt

1/4 tsp Cayenne Pepper

1 tsp Amino Acids (optional)

Directions

Run warm water over the spaghetti squash for a few minutes. Cut squash in half removing all seeds and membrane. Use a fork to scrape out the meat of the squash which should look noodle like. Add diced tomato onion, garlic and all seasonings to taste. Enjoy!

Easy Mashed Coconut Sweet Potatoes

4-5 large sweet potatoes

1/4 C coconut milk

2 tbsp unrefined coconut oil

1/2 tsp cinnamon

1/2 tsp sea salt

2 tbsp Agave nectar (optional)

Directions

Peel sweet potatoes and dice them into even pieces or you may leave them whole. Add them to a pot of water that comes just above the potatoes. Bring the potatoes to a boil and when they are fork tender you can remove them from the heat. You may use a potato masher or hand mixer to whip as you would mashed potatoes. Mix in all of the remaining ingredients and enjoy!

Rosemary-Garlic Mashed Potatoes

By Annette Hurt

4 cups chopped cauliflower

2 1/2 cups cashews, soaked for 1-2 hours

1/2 tsp himalayan salt

1-2 tsp chopped fresh rosemary

1 tsp minced garlic

2 tbsp white miso

2 tsp nutritional yeast

Directions

Place cauliflower in food processor, and process until it reaches a grain-like consistency. Add cashews, miso, and all other ingredients. Pulse in food processor to combine.

With processor running, add water in thin stream until mixture smooth whipped texture. For smoother texture place in vitamix or other blender with remaining ingredients and blend till combined.

Mushroom Gravy

By Annette Hurt

6 portabella mushroom caps

3 garlic cloves

3 tsptamari

3 tsp olive oil

1 cup walnuts

Directions

Soak walnuts for 30 min. Drain and rinse. Chop mushrooms into coarse pieces and place in blend. Add garlic, tamari, and walnuts. blend. Add water as needed for consistency. Drizzle in olive oil while blender is running. When gravy is smooth it is ready to serve.

Sunflower Nut Pate

By Nia Yaa

1 cup of walnuts or almonds

1/2 cup of sunflower seeds

1/4 cup chopped celery

1/4 cup chopped red onions

1/4 cup chopped bell pepper

2-4 cloves of garlic

2 tbsp. cold pressed olive oil

2 tbsp. amino acid or tamari sauce

Cumin, cayenne, spike to taste

Directions

Soak nuts and seeds with filtered or spring water overnight. Process nuts and seeds with a little water until they become smooth. Add the vegetables one at a time with other ingredients. Continue to process until you get a smooth texture. This pate is great wrapped in seaweed or green leaves.

Black Eye Pea Hummus

By Nia Yaa

1/4 bag of black eyed peas

3-5 garlic cloves

1/4 cup chopped red onions

1/4 cup of cold pressed olive oil

Soak peas overnight, rinse and discard the skins. Process all ingredients a little at a time until you get a smooth texture. Add sea salt to taste. Can be served with salt water crackers or tortilla chips.

Raw Chop Suey

By Nia Yaa

1/4 green cabbage

1/4 red cabbage

1/2 red onion

2 stalks celery

2 carrot

1/2 red bell pepper

1 cup of bean sprouts

2 cloves of garlic

1/4 cup of cold pressed olive oil

1/4 cup of sesame oil

1/3 cup of amino acid or tamari sauce

1/4 cup of rice vinegar

Directions

Slice all vegetables in thin strips, except for bean sprouts. Mix ingredients well and marinate for at least 4 hours before serving.

Affirmation: My body is a sacred temple.

Dorothy Jean's Tablespoon Cornbread

By Nova Kafele

First heat your stove to 350 degrees and in an iron skillet or 9 inch Pyrex baking dish put 1/2 cup of oil in the skillet and put it in the oven to heat while you get everything else together. Get your dry ingredients together.

In a medium size bowl measure:

8 heaping tablespoons of cornmeal

6 heaping tablespoons of kamut or amaranth flour. If you'd like you can do

3 & 3 of each.

Next, measure one level tablespoon of non aluminum baking powder.

Measure one half teaspoon of salt. Fold all that together. Then get your egg replacer together and mix enough to where it looks like the size of a real large egg or use 1 egg if you eat them. Put that over in the dry ingredients and then pour 3 cups rice or almond milk in the bowl. You don't want it too thick but a nice consistency.

Put about 1/2 cup of agave in the batter and blend well with your spoon. Now get your skillet with the oil and pour 2 tablespoons of oil in the batter and stir thoroughly. Then pour batter into hot skillet and this will give you a nice crust.

Bake at 350 degrees for about 40 minutes or until your knife comes out clean.

Cut it, butter it & be full of joy! Best with butter limas or purple hull peas, sweet potatoes and turnip greens! ;)

Sekhem Muffins (makes 12)

By Mut Shat Shemsut

1 cup organic dried apricots and figs or the organic dried fruit of your choice

1 cup coconut flour

¾ cup sweetener (If you must, try palm sugar, coconut sugar) OR, try the sweetness of the fruit only.

2 tbsp orange zest

1 cup organic pancake mix

½ tsp cinnamon

¼ tsp finely crushed Himalayan or other sea salt

¼ tsp baking powder OR 1 tsp organic apple cider vinegar (to help muffins rise)

1 cup of yogurt substitute such as coconut milk yogurt

Directions

Preheat oven to 350. Put water to boil. Place dried fruit in heatproof bowl. Cover with boiling water to plump up fruit, let stand 5 minutes, drain and set aside.

Coat stainless steel muffin pan with coconut oil. Combine coconut flour, pancake mix, sweetener, orange zest, and sea salt in a large wooden or glass bowl.

 Add fruit, and coconut milk yogurt in to the batter bowl. If the batter is too thick, add a little coconut or almond milk.

Fill muffin pans with batter, bake 20 to 25 minutes, then, insert toothpick into centers which should come out clean. Cool ten minutes in pan, remove

Affirmation: May this meal provide all that I need and remove that which I don't need.

Quinoa, Kidney Bean and Kale Salad

By Mut Shat Shemsut

2 cups cooked quinoa

1 ½ cups cooked kidney beans

1 cup grated carrots

½ cup hazelnuts, chopped

1 small red onion, thinly sliced

½ red bell pepper, chopped

½ orange bell pepper, chopped

3 cloves garlic, minced

1 tblsp turmeric powder (a cancer fighter)

2 tsp Bragg Liquid Aminos or the salt of your choice

Directions

Cook quinoa (15 minutes)

Place all other ingredients in a wooden or glass bowl and mix thoroughly. Add cooked quinoa and toss Kale, turnips, spinach, collards—help protect against retinal damage and the onset of cataracts and age-related macular degeneration.

Kidney Beans –full of zinc, a mineral helps get vitamin A from the liver to the retina which activates melanin production. Zinc helps with night vision, cataract prevention.

Quinoa (see page 52 for benefit details) lowers the glycemic-index which reduces the risk of age-related macular degeneration.

Note: Quinoa may be eaten raw as sprouts. However, if you're not going to carefully follow the steps on page 52, COOK IT!

Affirmation: May all who share in this meal be healthy, happy and whole.

Tasty Lentil Bean Soup

By Nia Yaa

1 bag of brown lentils

1/2 onion

1/2 chopped pepper

3 carrots

2 stalks of celery

1 can of coconut milk

1 tsp each of rosemary, thyme, cumin, curry, ginger

1 dash of sea salt

1 tbsp. of olive or sesame oil

2 cloves of garlic

1 habanero (optional)

Directions

Brown onion in oil in large pot. Then add beans and water. To cover the beans. Cook beans for 1/2 hour and add other ingredients. Add coconut milk, 1 more cup of water and habanero or other hot pepper to taste. Add a little more seasoning before serving.

Spicy Cabbage

By Nia Yaa

1/2 head cabbage

1/2 red onion

1/2 bell pepper

1/2 jalapeno pepper

2 tsp curry powder

Directions

Slice cabbage in thin strips and add to frying pan with a little olive oil. Add onion, pepper and spices. Add 1/2 cup of water, cover and simmer. Cook until cabbage becomes limp.

Vegan Gumbo

By Nia Yaa

1/2 lb of fried tofu

2 links of veggie sausage

1 red onion

1/2 green pepper

1/2 red pepper

3 stalks of celery

2 ears of corn

1/2 bag of black eye peas

2 carrots

3 red potatoes

1/2 lb string beans

1 large can of diced tomatoes

chili powder curry powder thyme, rosemary, parsley

Directions

In a large pot brown tofu and tofurkey sausage. Add onions, black eye peas, herbs and 6 cups of water. Cook for 1/2 hour then add vegetables one at a time. Add 1 large can of diced tomatoes, you may also need to add more water. Add spices and let cook for about 1 hour or until vegetables are soft.

Enjoy

*This is a heavy meal and can be made without the tofu and veggie sausage for a lighter version.

Affirmation: My hands prepare delicious and nutritious meals that the entire family can enjoy.

Spiced Curry Eggplant (Serves 4)

By Herb 'N Spice

Sprouted Organic Extra Firm Tofu

2 Asian (long, slender)Eggplants

2 tbsp Grape seed oil

½ med onion

4 Thai chili peppers

1-2 handfuls of curry leaves

Sea Salt

Green Life Spice Blend

1 tbsp coconut oil

1 tbsp white miso paste

Braggs Liquid Amino

Directions

Press and cube Sprouted Organic Extra Firm Tofu. Quarter and slice eggplant and soak in bowl of water with sea salt. Sautee tofu cubes in 2 tbsp. grape seed oil on med-high heat until browned. Stir and season with Green Life Spice Blend.

Remove Eggplant from salted water, drain and, add to pan. Add ½ med onion chopped, 4 Thai chili peppers (chopped) and add a handful (or two) curry leaves to the pan. Add 1 tbsp coconut oil, 1 tbsp. white miso paste and, stir fry ingredients. Add Braggs Liquid Amino to taste.

Affirmation: I give thanks for the fruits of the earth.

Curry Vegetables

By Nia Yaa

1/2 head of cabbage

3 red potatoes

3 carrots

2 stalks of celery

1/2 cup of onions

1 cup of peppers (green, red, or yellow)

2 tbsp. curry powder

1/2 cup tomato sauce

1/2 cup of water

1 tsp each of thyme, cumin, coriander, cayenne, ginger

Directions

Cut vegetables into chunks and warm olive oil in a large frying pan. Add cubed potatoes, and cook a few minuets. Then add onions, pepper, cabbage, carrots and mix well. Cook for about 5 minutes then add remaining ingredients.

Cook for about 30 minutes until vegetables are soft.

Serve with basmati or brown rice.

Affirmation: I heal my family with each meal.

Broccoli Tacos
By Nova Kafele

Start with 2 large broccoli crowns
1/2 cup corn (optional)
1/2 onion diced
2 garlic cloves minced
2 large green chilies roast over open fire of your stove eye or bake
1/2 tbsp cumin
1 tbsp chili powder
3 to 4 Tbsp olive oil for sauté'
1 1/2 tsp spike or 2 tbsp liquid aminos or add pink himalayan salt to taste

Directions

Steam broccoli uncovered so it won't lose its color and until tender. When cool, cut broccoli into desired size as to the way you want your taco filling to appear. Wash, dry and bake chilies at 350 degrees until tender and remove skins; roasting over the stove eye can be done as well which is the quicker way by just holding the chili by its stem and turning until the skin becomes black and chili becomes tender. Put over in a bowl and wait until cool enough to handle and remove the skins and seeds. Chop chills and set aside. Dice onions and garlic and put over in the skillet with olive oil and sauté' until the onions are tender. Once that is done fold all your ingredients over in that same pan with sautéed onions, garlic and add spices. Fold over with a wooden spoon and add a touch or two of hot boiling water to the ingredients. Fry yellow corn taco tortillas or warm them over the eye on your stove. Add shredded romaine, arugula or cabbage with tomato or salsa and enjoy! (Remember you can always add a little more of this or that to suit your taste.)

More on Elevation

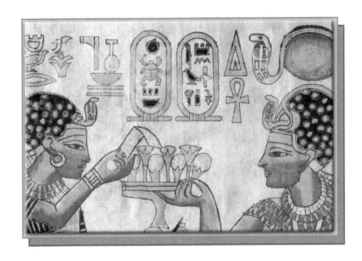

Boost Your Child's Brain Power!
By Mut Shat Shemsut

Parents don't consciously set out to starve their children's brains of nutrition. However, that is exactly what happens when children and teens are fed a steady diet of processed foods and sugars. As a retired school teacher whose career spanned almost three decades, I have observed a steady decline in cognitive function, commensurate, it appears, with increased consumption of non-nutritious foods. I observed an increased number of students who exhibited sluggishness, a lack of motivation, and an inability to process or retain information. Of course, other non-food related factors are involved, without question. However, the focus here is on food consumption. Though my observation was unscientific statistics and medical studies appear to confirm them.

Three Common Deficiencies in Children and Teens

According to Dr. David Suskind, Department of Pediatrics, Division of Pediatric Gastroenterology Hepatology and Nutrition, Seattle Children's Hospital, many children and teens that appear healthy may actually be nutrient deficient in ways that are negatively affecting them now and, I stress, could do so well into their academic futures. Dr. Suskind identified three of the most common nutrients lacking in otherwise healthy children and teens. They are iron, vitamin D3 and calcium/magnesium.

More info on the following chart.

Iron, Vitamin D3, Calcium/Magnesium Function and Deficiency Results	
Iron - Transports oxygen from the lungs to the tissues, muscles and *brain*. Essential for *immunity* and for *creating energy* from food.	Low energy, frequent illnesses, "foggy" brain. It is interesting to note that children/teens with ADD and ADHD are often low in iron.
Vitamin D3 - Essential for absorption of calcium in teeth, bones and muscle. Regulates hormones. Prevents cancer by promoting proper cell growth. Plays an essential role in *immunity* and *blood sugar regulation* and cardiovascular, muscle and *brain health*.	Vitamin D3 deficiencies tend to get worse as children age. Teens tend to be low in Vitamin D3 at a time when they need it most for hormonal regulation, immunity and mental processing.
Calcium/Magnesium - Building blocks of bones, teeth and soft tissue. Regulates muscle and nerve function and manage blood vessel contraction and dilation affecting blood pressure.	Hyperactivity, insomnia, anxiety, gum disease, muscle pains, and bones that are easily broken can be the result of calcium deficiency. At night, when the body slows down, children and teens may show the above symptoms, exhibiting anxiety, trouble sleeping, restless legs or unexplained pains.

You *Can* Boost Your Child's Brain Power

Plan your family meals in advance, providing foods that enrich the brain, and you can have an academic star whose potential is limitless!

Iron – organic vegetables, seeds, beans, grains, black-strap molasses. Dark green leafy vegetables, asparagus, green cabbage, green and red peppers, radishes, peas, broccoli, squash, cauliflower, Brussels sprouts and squash are iron-rich vegetables that also contain vitamin C. Vegetarians need vitamin C in order to easily absorb iron. Include lots of vitamin C containing fruit in the diet.

Vitamin D3 – Your body makes vitamin D3 when you expose it to the sun. Therefore, the sun is a natural source of this vitamin. Take time to sit in the sun, play in it, meditate in it—even do or oversee homework in it. According to The Vegetarian Resource Group, the most effective vitamin D sun exposure comes between the hours of 10 a.m. and 3 p.m. during summer months. Our skin is so intelligent that it stops producing vitamin D once we've had enough. Brown-skinned people, especially, need to ensure that intake of this vitamin are adequate, since brown pigmentation can block sun absorption. Other sources of vitamin D for vegetarians are white button mushrooms, foods fortified with vitamin D, such as cereal and D fortified, almond, oat, or hazelnut milk. Another source is supplements. The Vegetarian Resource Group has a list of vegan vitamin D supplements on its website.

Calcium – Kale, broccoli, collard greens, mustard greens, spinach, bok choy, almonds, oatmeal, molasses; oranges, tangerines, dried apricots, kiwi, dates, dried figs, prunes, mulberries, kumquats, prickly pears are all good sources of calcium.

Magnesium – Spinach, beet greens, okra, savoy cabbage, butternut squash, sweet corn, artichoke, peas, cucumber with peel; plantain, watermelon, raspberries, strawberries, kiwi, guava, jack fruit, grapefruit are all good sources of magnesium.

Staying Healthy as an Act of Revolution: What You Can Do

View taking ownership of the nutritional health of your children and your own health as an act of revolution. Shop on the outside aisles of supermarkets where the fruit and vegetables are stocked. Avoid the middle aisles laden with unhealthy processed foods. If you can't pronounce the words listing the ingredients—don't purchase it! Avoid pesticides, buy organic. Ensure that your children eat a healthy breakfast each morning. Research and find organic/vegetarian food buying clubs in your area. Attend vegetarian, vegan and raw food preparation workshops. If you can't find them, start one! Our health is truly our wealth and the path to a spiritual life as well.

References

Health. Alicious. Ness.com>. <http://www.healthaliciousness.com/articles/foods-high-in-magnesium.php>.

Livingstrong.com>. http://www.livestrong.com/article/212438-good-sources-of-calcium-for-vegetarians/>.

Vegetarian Resource Group. < http://www.vrg.org/journal/vj2009issue2/2009_issue2_vitamin_d.php>.

Suskind David L MD. Nutritional deficiencies during normal growth. Pediatric Clinics of North America, Volume 56, Issue 5, October 2009, Pages 1035-1053.

Affirmation: I receive all that I need for life, strength, and good health.

Fasting for Elevation

Fasting is something that should be done on a regular basis. There are many ways to fast. It is best to begin with a short fast and then build up to longer fasts, this will greatly improve your chances of success.

A day fast is a good start. Choose a day, give yourself 30 days to prepare if this is your first time. Fast from sun up to sun down. Drink only liquid, filtered water, tea or lemon water. Eat a light meal at sundown, salad and fruit is best. If you overeat you will limit the benefit of the fast.

A 24 hour liquid fast is also a good place to start to build up your discipline. You can choose a day of the week, for instance Friday, have a meal on Thursday eve and 7 and then eat again Friday and 7pm. Once again when you break your fast it is important to eat light and do not consume drugs or alcohol. Drink only filtered water and herbal tea. You may also want to add lemon, chlorophyll or spirulina to your water for extra energy and nutrition. Next try a 3 day, 7 day, 14, 21 or even 40 day fast for maximum benefit.

Another popular way to fast is a raw food fast. One would eat 75% to 100 % raw fruit, veggies, nuts, seeds, fresh juices and purified water. This is perfect for those who work long hours and need to have energy during the daytime. A raw food fast could be 1 or 100 days. If you are over 30 and have not taken time to truly detox your body, you may want to choose to fast for 30 or more days to give your body an opportunity to restart and clear for your next 30 years.

Your fast is up to you , if you are a meat eater, you may want to start with fasting from meat, junk food and fast food. You may need to fast from soda or sugar water drinks. Remember you fast to give your body an opportunity to rest and clear toxins that it cannot clear when it is digesting food all day every day.

You may also find it helpful to fast from TV and other electronic devices. A talk fast can be helpful when you are having trouble communicating. Of course fasting from anything that is not serving your highest good is suggested.

While fasting try to remain peaceful, still and quiet as much as possible. While your body is resting you are more open to the messages of Spirit. You may also find it helpful to wear white or light clothes to reflect your time of cleansing. Choose to be alone or with others who are fasting, to minimize the challenges when others around you are having meals.

Listen to spiritual or uplifting music, read positive books, or write in your journal to receive the greatest benefits of your fast. While you fast physically, you will also notice a change in your mental and emotional states as well.

You may feel like crying or releasing energy, you may be full of energy and looking for new outlets to use it. Other reactions may be headaches, nausea, restlessness, etc. These symptoms are common when your body begins to release toxins. Drinking water, exercise, sauna, soaking in Epsom salt and colon therapy are ways to assist your body in releasing toxins.

When you stop eating your digestion process will slow down. Using herbs such as aloe vera and cascara sagrada will assist your body in releasing accumulated waste. Clearing the waste from your colon will allow your blood to be more alkaline and for your body to absorb vital nutrients into your blood as well.

Fasting can add years to your life and overall higher quality of health and wellness. Fasting will increase your will and your discipline. Fasting will also enhance your spiritual connection and your spiritual powers.

Nia Yaa

Excerpt from Body Type Analysis Guide by MediaPower

Each body is different due to biochemical reactions. Your body is composed of a series of biochemical reactions that help it function properly. Chemical reactions cannot occur in the body without enzymes.

Each Body Type has specific enzyme needs. Vitamins, minerals and hormones cannot carry out their jobs without enzymes and the body cannot function without enzymes, as they are catalysts necessary for good health.

There are four Body Types that can be linked to specific enzyme deficiencies:

Body Type 1 people have shoulders and hips that are about the same width and frequently have an hourglass figure. When these people gain weight, it spreads throughout their body, causing an increase in overall size. Excess weight is held in their stomach and hips. They are prone to low blood pressure, allergies, cold hands/feet, and depression and mood swings.

Type 1 people are carbohydrate lovers and crave foods such as pastas, breads, desserts, butter and jam. This leads them to become deficient in Amylase, the enzyme that breaks down excess carbohydrates and sugars, which leads to improper digestion and unhealthful cravings, hypoglycemia, anxiety, fatigue, and inflammation.

Body Type 2 people have narrow shoulders and wider hips, often described as a 'pear figure'. When these people gain weight, it settles first in their hips, stomach, and butt. They are prone to cysts and skin disorders, indigestion, gallbladder issues, and kidney and bladder infections.

Type 2 people crave foods rich in flavor and high in fats such as fried, creamy, and spicy foods and desserts. This leads them to become deficient in Lipase, the enzyme that digests fats, which leads to undigested fats, high cholesterol levels, high blood pressure and stress on the liver.

Body Type 3 people have shoulders wider than their hips and frequently have a "cone-shaped" figure. While their legs remain strong well into old age, their weight gain tends to settle first in their upper torso and then their hips.

Type 3 people crave protein such as red meats, fish, poultry, nuts, cheese, eggs and salty foods. This can lead to deficiency in Protease, causing more protein cravings. They are prone to undigested protein in the colon area leading to the undigested matter being resorbed back into the body, blood, muscles, joints, lymphatic system and skin.

Body Type 4 people have small figures and soft bodies, often described as a "stick-figure". They have a sensitive and fragile Body Type prone to toxicity; If they gain weight, it is spread evenly and looks like baby fat.

Type 4 people crave dairy such as milk, yogurt, cream cheese, starchy foods and sweets. They often develop a deficiency in Lactase, the enzyme that breaks down dairy products and milk sugars. They are prone to on-going bowel problems, constipation and diarrhea, skin irritation, sinus infections, and nausea after eating. They have trouble digesting fiber and fats, which can lead to poor nutrition.

A lack of enzymes, or a deficiency in a particular enzyme, will significantly affect the function of the body. Having good nutrition and a chemically balanced body is vitally important as a large supply of enzymes in the body are allocated to the digestive system and help break down foods we eat and transport nutrients into the blood stream for assimilation and use by the cells.

Meet the Authors

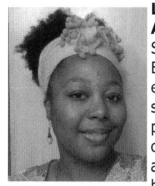

Lauren Markham aka Aqseshsha Asu-At was born and raised in South Bend, IN. She attended the University of Alabama at Birmingham where she acquired her bachelors in Foreign Language with an emphasis in Spanish. Her love for culture and people led her to the healing arts and a certification as a Kemetic Reiki practitioner and master teacher since 2012. Ra Sekhi has been influential and life changing in all areas including diet. Since becoming a practitioner she has lost a little over 30 pounds and counting which she directly attributes to adhering to the Ra Sekhi principles and practices. An advocate for womb health, she is also a part of the Yoni Steam Institute as a certified yoni steam practitioner and womb yoga instructor. She also specializes in diagnostic facial reading, aromatherapy, and color therapy. She is available for consultation and treatments at the Vibrance Center in South Bend, IN.

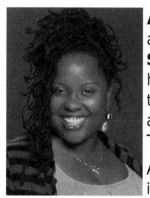

Aura Agape is a wholistic wellness consultant and product developer of **Herbs'N Spice, LLC.** She has been a long-time herbologist, herbalist and a holistic practitioner with a degree in Agriculture. Aura is an ordained minister, Kemetic Reiki Master Teacher & Holistic Doula.

Aura's scope of knowledge and experience is in various plant cultivation and soil conservation techniques, aromatherapy, herbal preparations and foods that heal. Much of her research and the articles she has written are in regard to holistic approaches to healing, wellness, and life. Aura creates natural products for the home and body in which their uses range from culinary to therapeutic. She has the passion and knowledge to spread the message and consciousness that we are already armed with the right tools to live a life of wellness and to overcome our perceived problems.

Aura takes a stand to advocate the rights of individuals to make informed choices in regard to individual and family health. As an innovative educator of healing foods, herbs and preparation techniques, Aura's goal is to empower you to take responsibility of your own health, activities and resources.

For more information regarding products, services or, to set up an appointment for consultation www.herbnspicewellness.com

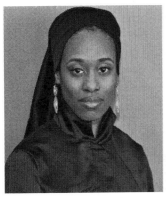 **Qamarah Muhammad El Shamesh** was attuned to Usui Reiki Level I in 2009 and Usui Reiki Level II in 2010. In 2011, she began her year of Reiki Master training in both Usui Reiki & Ra Sekhi Kemetic Reiki. She is certified in Ra Sekhi Kemetic Reiki Levels 1&2 and holds a Level 3 Ra Sekhi Master Level Teacher Certification and Usui Reiki.

In describing what becoming a Ra Sekhi Kemetic Reiki Master means to her, Qamarah reflects that the master attunement was a big step that allowed her to take a deeper look at her life purpose as it continues to inspire her to make healing work a daily part of her life. It sprang from a sincere desire to help others as well as to develop and express important virtues like compassion, cooperation and kindness. This path required deep self study and meditation on Universal Life Force energy and continues to be a journey that fosters in her an outpouring of love and understanding for those around her.

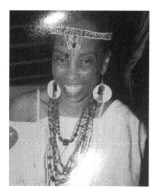

Rekhit Kajara Nia Yaa Nebthet an author, healer, priestess, teacher, artist and founder of the Ra Sekhi Arts Temple. She has dedicated her life to heal and uplift people by promoting health and wellness in the community. She is available for classes, consultations and presentations.

Email rasekhitemple@gmail.com

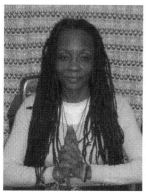

Mut Shat Shemsut/Gianprem is a Level 2 practitioner of Ra Sekhi Kemetic Reiki, having studied with Master Teacher Rekhit Kajara Nebthet in Oakland, California. She is also a certified Kundalini Yoga teacher. After eight years of practice, she began study with Krishna Kaur in Los Angeles, receiving her Level 1 certification in 2008. Level 2 certifications were acquired under lead trainer Gurucharan Singh Khalsa in Espanola, New Mexico and at Kundalini Yoga East in New York, with Sat Jivan Singh and Sat Jivan Kaur. She is a certified Y.O.G. A. for Youth teacher. Mut Shat gives her clients the benefit of both transforming modalities, assigning personalized Kundalini yoga meditations to address individual needs as determined by the Kemetic reiki sessions. She sees clients at her Bronx location, *In Light Yoga and Health.* Mut Shat Shemsut is a *Sacred Woman* (Queen Afua) and Member of African Holistic Health Chapter, New York. She is a retired public school educator.

Contact:
In Light Yoga and Health
Bronx, New York
www.inlightyogaandhealth.com
inlightyoga@earthlink.net

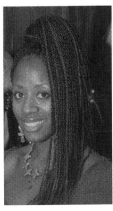

Empress Tabia "Khet Ra Maat" aka Eyiwtns Sol was born and raised to question and ask why? There isn't anything that will constrain her that isn't self-imposed. Her mission is healing thru word, organizing, energy exchange, touch and laying on of the hands.

She is a scholar who turned a B.A. in Psychology into the tool that has transformed her view of life. She is currently practicing Massage Therapy and is certified in Pre and Perinatal Massage, Womb Health and Wisdom/ Sacred Woman Training from the renowned Queen Afua, and a Kemetic Reiki practitioner of the Ra Sekhi Arts Temple. She is launching her business 'Empressive Healing' in the Spring of 2014! Life is beautiful and continues to blossom and she invites you to join her on the road to Wellness.

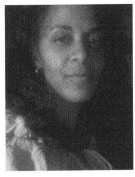

Nova Kafele-Lilly is a Mother of three Children and one grand daughter. I was raised in Compton, California to Claude and Dorothy Burch. I have two brothers, Lloyd and Mark and one sister, Peyton. The baby out of the bunch I guess one could say, that I came at a time where my parents consciousness was at its peak and greatest for they raised me in metaphysical and science of mind teachings. I am a Healer, Birthworker, community activist, farmer and produce purveyor, feminine health practitioner, teacher and wife to Jemal Lilly, my life partner and soul mate, and partner and owner of KRSTMoor Produce. We provide produce to communities in two counties, San Bernardino and Los Angeles.

We appreciate your support and pray this work will be a blessing to you. For more info about Ra Sekhi Arts Temple

visit us online

www.rasekhistore.com

www.rasekhihealing.com

www.rasekhi.bandcamp.com

www.youtube.com/rasekhiartstemple

Email: recipes4elevation@gmail.com

You can also like us on Facebook, Twitter and Instagram

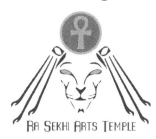

Made in the USA
Charleston, SC
02 February 2015